CKD Stage 3 and Diabetes Type 2 Cookbook

Relishing in Flavorful Cuisine: Delectable Recipes Catering to Diabetes and CKD Stage 3 Needs

McDonnell B. Young

Copyright © 2024 by **McDonnell B. Young**
All rights reserved

No part of this publication may be reproduced, stored in a retrieval system, or transmitted, in any form or by any means, electronic, mechanical, photocopying, recording, or otherwise, without the prior written permission of the author.

The information in this ebook is true and complete to the best of our knowledge. All recommendation are made without guarantee on the part of author or publisher. The author and publisher disclaim any liability in connection with the use of this information.

Table of Contents

Introduction	4
Understanding CKD and Diabetes	8
The Importance of a Healthy Diet	11
How to Use This Cookbook	14
Chapter 1: Breakfast Recipes	17
Oatmeal with Fresh Berries	17
Scrambled Eggs with Spinach	19
Greek Yogurt with Chia Seeds	21
Whole Grain Toast with Avocado	23
Smoothie with Kale and Almond Milk	25
Cottage Cheese with Pineapple	27
Blueberry Muffins (Low-Sugar)	29
Tofu Scramble with Veggies	32
Quinoa Porridge with Almonds	34
Apple Cinnamon Overnight Oats	36
Chapter 2: Lunch Recipes	38
Grilled Chicken Salad	38
Quinoa and Black Bean Bowl	41
Lentil Soup with Vegetables	43
Turkey and Avocado Wrap	45
Chickpea Salad with Cucumber	47
Spinach and Feta Stuffed Peppers	49
Broccoli and Cheese Quiche (Low-Sodium)	51

Tuna Salad with Olive Oil Dressing	53
Baked Salmon with Asparagus	55
Veggie Stir-Fry with Tofu	57
Chapter 3: Dinner Recipes	**59**
Baked Chicken with Rosemary	59
Beef and Vegetable Stew	61
Grilled Shrimp with Zucchini Noodles	63
Stuffed Bell Peppers with Quinoa	65
Eggplant Parmesan (Low-Sodium)	68
Roasted Turkey Breast with Brussels Sprouts	71
Pork Tenderloin with Apples	73
Spaghetti Squash with Tomato Sauce	75
Cod Fillet with Green Beans	77
Chickpea and Spinach Curry	79
Chapter 4: Snacks and Desserts	**81**
Healthy Snack Options	81
Healthy Dessert Options	82
Diabetes-Friendly Desserts	85
Conclusion	**90**

Introduction

As the sun set over the bustling city, a soft golden light filtered through the kitchen window of Sarah Thompson's cozy apartment. Sarah, a spirited woman in her mid-fifties, had spent the last few months adjusting to a new reality—living with Chronic Kidney Disease (CKD) Stage 3 and Type 2 Diabetes. Life had thrown her a curveball, but Sarah was determined to navigate this journey with grace and resilience.

It all started when Sarah began experiencing unusual fatigue and persistent thirst. A visit to her doctor revealed the diagnosis that changed her life. With a firm resolve to manage her health, Sarah began researching ways to live well with her conditions. That's when she stumbled upon the "CKD Stage 3 and Diabetes Type 2 Cookbook."

Intrigued by the promise of tailored recipes designed to support kidney function and maintain blood sugar levels, Sarah decided to give the guide a try. From the moment she opened the cookbook, she felt a sense of hope and empowerment. The introduction spoke directly to her, offering not just recipes but a comprehensive approach to managing her health.

The cookbook began with an enlightening overview of CKD Stage 3 and Type 2 Diabetes, explaining how the two conditions interlinked and the importance of a balanced diet. It was written in a warm, conversational tone, making complex medical information easy to understand. Sarah appreciated the friendly advice on portion control, the significance of choosing the right ingredients, and the impact of various nutrients on her health.

The first section, dedicated to breakfast recipes, was a revelation. Sarah discovered delicious and easy-to-prepare options like "Blueberry Chia Pudding" and "Spinach and Mushroom Omelette." Each recipe was carefully crafted to include ingredients that were gentle on her kidneys and helped maintain stable blood sugar levels. The nutritional breakdown provided with each dish reassured Sarah that she was making informed choices.

Moving on to lunch options, Sarah found a delightful variety of meals that were both satisfying and nutritious. The "Grilled Chicken and Quinoa Salad" quickly became her favorite. It was packed with lean protein and fiber, perfect for her dietary needs. The cookbook emphasized the importance of low-sodium ingredients, helping Sarah keep her blood pressure in check while enjoying flavorful meals.

Dinner time was no longer a challenge with the cookbook's array of hearty and wholesome recipes. The "Baked Salmon with Asparagus" was a standout, offering a rich source of omega-3 fatty acids beneficial for both her kidneys and heart. Sarah appreciated the detailed instructions and tips on meal preparation, making her feel like a confident chef in her own kitchen.

Beyond the recipes, the cookbook included invaluable tips and strategies for meal planning and grocery shopping. Sarah learned how to read food labels effectively, choose the best substitutes for high-phosphorus and high-potassium foods, and incorporate more fresh produce into her diet. The practical advice on managing portion sizes and staying hydrated became essential parts of her daily routine.

One of the most heartwarming aspects of the cookbook was the personal stories and testimonials from others living with CKD and Type 2 Diabetes. Reading about their journeys, challenges, and successes made Sarah feel connected and supported. She realized she wasn't alone in her struggle and that many had found a path to better health through the guidance of this cookbook.

As weeks turned into months, Sarah noticed significant improvements in her overall well-being. Her energy levels increased, her blood sugar levels stabilized, and her kidney function tests showed positive progress. She felt more vibrant and in control of her health than ever before.

Sarah often found herself recommending the "CKD Stage 3 and Diabetes Type 2 Cookbook" to friends and family. She would passionately explain how it wasn't just a collection of recipes but a comprehensive guide to living well with chronic conditions. The cookbook had become her trusted companion, offering not just nourishment but hope and inspiration.

In the quiet moments of reflection, Sarah realized that investing in the cookbook was one of the best decisions she had ever made. It had transformed her kitchen into a haven of health and wellness, empowering her to take charge of her life with confidence and joy.

If you're navigating the complexities of CKD Stage 3 and Type 2 Diabetes, Sarah's story is a testament to the profound impact the "CKD Stage 3 and Diabetes Type 2 Cookbook" can have on your journey. It's more than just a guide; it's a lifeline to better health and a brighter future.

Understanding CKD and Diabetes

Understanding CKD and Diabetes is essential for anyone living with these conditions, especially when it comes to managing diet and lifestyle. Chronic Kidney Disease (CKD) and Type 2 Diabetes are two interconnected health issues that require careful attention and management. CKD Stage 3 signifies moderate kidney damage, which impacts the kidneys' ability to filter waste and fluids effectively. On the other hand, Type 2 Diabetes affects how the body processes blood sugar, leading to potential complications in various organs, including the kidneys. Therefore, a comprehensive approach to diet is crucial for managing both conditions simultaneously.

The CKD Stage 3 and Diabetes Type 2 Cookbook provides a detailed understanding of how to balance nutrition to support kidney function and maintain blood sugar levels. This cookbook emphasizes the importance of choosing foods that are low in sodium, potassium, and phosphorus, which are essential for kidney health. By selecting the right ingredients, individuals can help prevent further kidney damage and reduce the risk of complications. The cookbook offers practical tips and recipes that are not only kidney-friendly but also effective in managing diabetes.

Dietary recommendations for CKD Stage 3 and Type 2 Diabetes often overlap, creating a unique set of guidelines that need to be followed. The CKD Stage 3 and Diabetes Type 2 Cookbook highlights the importance of consuming lean proteins, whole grains, and fresh vegetables while avoiding processed foods high in sodium and sugar. This balanced approach helps in controlling blood sugar levels and reduces the strain on the kidneys. Additionally, the cookbook provides alternatives and substitutes for common high-potassium and high-phosphorus foods, making it easier to plan meals that are both healthy and satisfying.

One of the critical aspects of managing CKD and Diabetes is portion control. Overeating can lead to weight gain, which exacerbates both conditions. The CKD Stage 3 and Diabetes Type 2 Cookbook includes portion control tips and strategies to help individuals maintain a healthy weight. By following these guidelines, people can enjoy a variety of delicious meals without compromising their health. The cookbook's focus on balanced, nutrient-dense meals ensures that individuals get the necessary vitamins and minerals without overloading their kidneys or spiking their blood sugar levels.

Fluid management is another important factor in managing CKD Stage 3 and Diabetes. The kidneys' reduced ability to filter waste means that fluid intake must be monitored carefully. The CKD Stage 3 and Diabetes Type 2 Cookbook provides guidance on how to stay hydrated without overburdening the kidneys. It includes recipes for beverages that are safe and beneficial for individuals with CKD and Diabetes, such as infused water and herbal teas. These drink options help maintain hydration while supporting overall kidney function.

Incorporating the right types of fats into the diet is also crucial for managing CKD and Diabetes. The CKD Stage 3 and Diabetes Type 2 Cookbook emphasizes the importance of healthy fats, such as those found in fish, nuts, and seeds. These fats help reduce inflammation and improve heart health, which is vital for individuals with both CKD and Diabetes. By including recipes that are rich in omega-3 fatty acids and other healthy fats, the cookbook ensures that individuals can enjoy flavorful meals that support their overall health.

Living with CKD Stage 3 and Type 2 Diabetes requires a comprehensive approach to diet and lifestyle. The CKD Stage 3 and Diabetes Type 2 Cookbook serves as a valuable resource, offering practical advice, delicious recipes, and a thorough understanding of how to manage these conditions effectively. By following the guidance provided in the cookbook, individuals can take control of their health, improve their quality of life, and prevent further complications. The cookbook is not just about food; it's about fostering a healthier, more balanced way of living that empowers individuals to thrive despite their diagnoses.

The Importance of a Healthy Diet

A healthy diet is paramount for individuals living with CKD Stage 3 and Type 2 Diabetes. The delicate balance required to manage both conditions can be achieved through thoughtful food choices that support kidney function and maintain stable blood sugar levels. By understanding the intricate relationship between these two health issues and diet, one can take significant steps toward better health and improved quality of life.

Foods low in sodium, phosphorus, and potassium are essential for individuals with CKD Stage 3. Excessive intake of these elements can burden the kidneys, leading to further deterioration of kidney function. Incorporating fresh fruits and vegetables, lean proteins, and whole grains into daily meals helps manage these mineral levels. Simultaneously, these foods offer the necessary nutrients to keep the body nourished without overworking the kidneys.

Managing Type 2 Diabetes requires consistent control of blood sugar levels. This is best achieved through a diet rich in fiber, healthy fats, and lean proteins while minimizing refined sugars and carbohydrates. Balanced meals that include complex carbohydrates, such as those found in whole grains, alongside proteins and healthy fats, ensure that blood sugar levels remain stable throughout the day. This approach not only helps in controlling diabetes but also supports overall metabolic health.

The recipes in the CKD Stage 3 and Diabetes Type 2 Cookbook are meticulously designed to meet these dietary needs. Each recipe is crafted with ingredients that are beneficial for both kidney health and blood sugar management. For instance, dishes featuring fish like salmon or trout provide omega-3 fatty acids, which are heart-healthy and support inflammation reduction. Paired with low-potassium vegetables, these meals become powerful tools in maintaining overall health.

Hydration plays a crucial role in managing both CKD and diabetes. Proper fluid intake helps the kidneys filter waste more effectively and keeps the body hydrated, which is essential for all metabolic processes. The cookbook includes tips on how to stay hydrated without overconsumption, ensuring that fluid balance is maintained. Drinking adequate water, herbal teas, and other kidney-friendly beverages can make a significant difference in how one feels daily.

Portion control is another critical aspect highlighted in the cookbook. Overeating can lead to weight gain and elevated blood sugar levels, which exacerbate both kidney disease and diabetes. The recipes provide clear guidelines on portion sizes, helping individuals avoid excess caloric intake while ensuring they receive sufficient nutrients. This practice not only aids in weight management but also enhances the efficacy of the dietary plan.

Meal planning and preparation are key strategies emphasized in the CKD Stage 3 and Diabetes Type 2 Cookbook. By planning meals in advance, individuals can ensure they have access to healthy, balanced options throughout the week. This reduces the temptation to reach for convenient, processed foods that are often high in sodium and sugars. The cookbook provides practical advice on meal prepping, grocery shopping, and organizing the kitchen to make healthy eating more manageable.

Incorporating a healthy diet tailored to the needs of CKD Stage 3 and Type 2 Diabetes can lead to remarkable improvements in overall health and well-being. By following the comprehensive dietary guidance offered in the cookbook, individuals can take proactive steps toward managing their conditions effectively. The benefits extend beyond physical health, fostering a sense of control and empowerment in one's health journey.

How to Use This Cookbook

When you first open the CKD Stage 3 and Diabetes Type 2 Cookbook, you'll find that it is more than just a collection of recipes; it's a comprehensive guide designed to support your health journey. Begin by familiarizing yourself with the initial sections that provide a clear understanding of how CKD Stage 3 and Type 2 Diabetes interact. These sections explain the importance of diet in managing both conditions and offer valuable insights into how the right food choices can make a significant difference in your health.

As you dive into the recipes, notice that each one is meticulously crafted to balance the nutritional needs of individuals with CKD and Type 2 Diabetes. Pay close attention to the ingredient lists and preparation methods, which are designed to limit sodium, potassium, and phosphorus intake while providing ample protein and fiber. The nutritional information provided with each recipe will help you understand how each dish fits into your daily dietary requirements, making it easier to plan your meals effectively.

The cookbook also includes practical advice on meal planning and portion control, which are crucial for managing both CKD and diabetes. You'll find tips on how to create a balanced meal plan that accommodates your dietary restrictions without sacrificing flavor or variety. This section encourages you to plan your meals ahead of time, ensuring that you always have healthy options available, even on your busiest days.

Shopping for ingredients can be a daunting task, but the cookbook simplifies this process with detailed guidelines on what to look for in the grocery store. Learn how to read food labels to avoid high-sodium and high-potassium items, and discover healthier alternatives to common ingredients that might be detrimental to your health. This will make your shopping trips more efficient and help you make better choices that align with your dietary needs.

In addition to the recipes, the cookbook provides strategies for dining out and handling social situations where food is involved. It offers advice on how to make smart choices when eating at restaurants and how to communicate your dietary needs to others. These tips are designed to empower you to maintain your dietary regimen without feeling deprived or isolated from social activities.

Another important aspect of this cookbook is its focus on hydration and fluid management, which are critical for those with CKD. You will find information on how much fluid you should consume daily and tips on staying hydrated without exceeding your limits. The recipes also include suggestions for beverages that are safe and beneficial for your condition, ensuring you stay properly hydrated throughout the day.

Finally, the cookbook includes personal stories and testimonials from others who have successfully managed CKD and Type 2 Diabetes with the help of this guide. These stories offer inspiration and practical advice, showing you that it is possible to live a full and healthy life despite these conditions. By following the recipes and tips in this cookbook, you will be well on your way to better managing your health and improving your overall quality of life.

Chapter 1: Breakfast Recipes

Oatmeal with Fresh Berries

Ingredients:
- 1/2 cup rolled oats
- 1 cup water or low-fat milk
- 1/4 teaspoon salt (optional)
- 1/2 cup fresh berries (blueberries, strawberries, raspberries)
- 1 tablespoon ground flaxseed
- 1/4 teaspoon cinnamon (optional)
- Sugar substitute or honey (to taste, optional)

Instructions:
1. In a small saucepan, bring water or milk to a boil. Add the rolled oats and salt, and stir.
2. Reduce heat and simmer for 5 minutes, stirring occasionally, until the oats are soft and have absorbed most of the liquid.
3. Remove from heat and let it sit for 2 minutes to thicken further.

4. Stir in the ground flaxseed and cinnamon. Sweeten with a sugar substitute or honey if desired.

5. Serve in a bowl and top with fresh berries.

Nutritional Information (per serving):

- Calories: 200
- Protein: 6 g
- Carbohydrates: 38 g
- Fiber: 6 g
- Sugar: 7 g (natural sugars from berries)
- Fat: 3 g
- Sodium: 120 mg (without added salt)

Serving Size: 1 bowl

Cooking Time: 10 minutes

Scrambled Eggs with Spinach

Ingredients:

- 2 large eggs
- 1 cup fresh spinach, chopped
- 1 tablespoon olive oil
- Salt and pepper to taste (optional)
- 1 tablespoon low-fat cheese, shredded (optional)

Instructions:

1. Heat the olive oil in a non-stick skillet over medium heat.
2. Add the chopped spinach to the skillet and sauté for 2-3 minutes, or until the spinach is wilted.
3. In a bowl, whisk the eggs with salt and pepper if using. Pour the eggs over the wilted spinach.
4. Allow the eggs to sit undisturbed for about a minute, then gently stir with a spatula, lifting and folding it over from the bottom to let the uncooked eggs flow underneath.
5. Sprinkle shredded cheese over the eggs, if using, and cook for another minute or until the eggs are fully cooked but still soft and fluffy.
6. Remove from heat and serve immediately.

Nutritional Information:
- Calories: 215
- Total Fat: 16g
- Saturated Fat: 4g
- Cholesterol: 372mg
- Sodium: 220mg (note: adding salt will change this)
- Total Carbohydrates: 2g
- Dietary Fiber: 1g
- Sugars: 1g
- Protein: 14g

Serving Size:
- Serves 1

Cooking Time:
- Prep time: 5 minutes
- Cook time: 6 minutes

Greek Yogurt with Chia Seeds

Ingredients:

- 1 cup plain Greek yogurt (low-fat)
- 2 tablespoons chia seeds
- 1/2 cup fresh blueberries
- 1 tablespoon almond slices
- 1 teaspoon honey (optional, for sweetness)

Instructions:

1. In a serving bowl, combine the Greek yogurt and chia seeds. Stir thoroughly until the chia seeds are evenly distributed.
2. Gently fold in the fresh blueberries and almond slices into the yogurt mixture.
3. If desired, drizzle honey over the mixture for added sweetness. This step is optional and should be used sparingly for those monitoring their sugar intake.
4. Refrigerate the mixture for at least 30 minutes, allowing the chia seeds to swell and absorb some of the yogurt, thickening the texture slightly.
5. Serve chilled.

Nutritional Information (per serving):

- Calories: 180
- Total Fat: 4g
- Saturated Fat: 1g
- Cholesterol: 5mg
- Sodium: 55mg
- Total Carbohydrates: 19g
- Dietary Fiber: 4g
- Sugars: 12g (includes 1g added sugars from honey)
- Protein: 16g

Serving Size: 1 bowl (approximately 1.5 cups)

Cooking Time: No cooking required; refrigerate for at least 30 minutes.

Whole Grain Toast with Avocado

Ingredients:
- 2 slices of whole grain bread
- 1 ripe avocado
- Pinch of salt (optional)
- Ground black pepper (to taste)
- 1 teaspoon of lemon juice

Instructions:
1. Toast the whole grain bread slices to your desired level of crispiness.
2. While the bread is toasting, peel and pit the avocado. In a small bowl, mash the avocado with a fork until it reaches a smooth consistency.
3. Add lemon juice, a pinch of salt (if using), and black pepper to the mashed avocado. Mix well.
4. Spread the avocado mixture evenly on the toasted bread slices.
5. Serve immediately.

Nutritional Information:
- Calories: 210 per serving

- Total Fat: 12g
- Saturated Fat: 2g
- Cholesterol: 0mg
- Sodium: 180mg
- Total Carbohydrates: 24g
- Dietary Fiber: 7g
- Sugars: 3g
- Protein: 5g

Serving Size:
1 serving consists of 2 avocado toasts.

Cooking Time:
Preparation time: 5 minutes
Cook time: 3 minutes

Smoothie with Kale and Almond Milk

Ingredients:

- 1 cup fresh kale, chopped
- 1 cup unsweetened almond milk
- 1/2 green apple, cored and chopped
- 1 tablespoon chia seeds
- 1/2 teaspoon ground cinnamon
- 1/4 avocado
- Ice cubes (optional, for thicker consistency)

Instructions:

1. Rinse the kale leaves thoroughly under cold water to remove any dirt or debris.
2. In a blender, combine the chopped kale, almond milk, chopped green apple, chia seeds, ground cinnamon, and avocado.
3. Add a few ice cubes if a thicker consistency is desired.
4. Blend on high speed until smooth and creamy, approximately 1-2 minutes, ensuring all components are fully incorporated.
5. Taste and adjust the smoothness by adding more almond milk if necessary.
6. Serve immediately for the best flavor and nutrient retention.

Nutritional Information (per serving):

- Calories: 180
- Protein: 4 grams
- Fat: 8 grams
- Carbohydrates: 24 grams
- Fiber: 6 grams
- Sugar: 11 grams
- Sodium: 95 mg

Serving Size: 1 serving (approximately 1 1/2 cups)

Cooking Time: 5 minutes

Cottage Cheese with Pineapple

Ingredients:
- 1/2 cup low-fat cottage cheese
- 1/2 cup fresh pineapple, chopped
- 1 tablespoon chopped almonds (optional)
- 1 teaspoon ground flaxseed (optional)
- Fresh mint for garnish (optional)

Instructions:
1. In a serving bowl, place the cottage cheese.
2. Top the cottage cheese with freshly chopped pineapple.
3. If desired, sprinkle chopped almonds and ground flaxseed over the top for added texture and nutritional benefits.
4. Garnish with fresh mint leaves for a refreshing touch.
5. Serve immediately or chill in the refrigerator for 10 minutes before serving if preferred chilled.

Nutritional Information:
- Calories: 180 kcal
- Protein: 14 g
- Carbohydrates: 15 g

- Fat: 6 g
- Sodium: 350 mg
- Fiber: 2 g
- Sugar: 12 g

Serving Size: 1 serving

Cooking Time: 5 minutes (Preparation time)

Blueberry Muffins (Low-Sugar)

Ingredients:

- 1 ½ cups almond flour
- ½ cup oat bran
- ¼ cup stevia or your preferred sugar substitute
- 1 tsp baking powder
- ½ tsp baking soda
- ¼ tsp salt
- 2 large eggs
- ¼ cup unsweetened almond milk
- ¼ cup unsweetened applesauce
- 1 tsp vanilla extract
- 1 cup fresh blueberries

Instructions:

1. Preheat your oven to 350°F (175°C). Line a muffin tin with paper liners or grease with non-stick cooking spray.
2. In a large bowl, whisk together the almond flour, oat bran, stevia, baking powder, baking soda, and salt.
3. In another bowl, beat the eggs lightly and mix in the almond milk, applesauce, and vanilla extract until well combined.

4. Add the wet ingredients to the dry ingredients, stirring until just combined. Gently fold in the blueberries.
5. Spoon the batter into the prepared muffin tin, filling each cup about three-quarters full.
6. Bake in the preheated oven for 20-25 minutes, or until a toothpick inserted into the center of a muffin comes out clean.
7. Allow the muffins to cool in the pan for 5 minutes before transferring them to a wire rack to cool completely.

Nutritional Information (per serving):
- Calories: 140
- Protein: 6g
- Fat: 10g
- Carbohydrates: 8g
- Fiber: 3g
- Sugar: 2g

Serving Size:
- Makes 12 muffins
- Serving size: 1 muffin

Cooking Time:
- Preparation time: 10 minutes

- Cooking time: 20-25 minutes
- Total time: 30-35 minutes

Tofu Scramble with Veggies

Ingredients:

- 8 oz firm tofu, drained and crumbled
- 1 tbsp olive oil
- 1/2 red bell pepper, diced
- 1/2 green bell pepper, diced
- 1 small onion, finely chopped
- 1 cup chopped spinach
- 1/2 tsp turmeric
- 1/4 tsp black pepper
- 1/4 tsp salt (optional, adjust based on dietary needs)
- 1/2 tsp garlic powder
- 1 tbsp nutritional yeast (for a cheesy flavor)

Instructions:

1. Heat the olive oil in a non-stick skillet over medium heat.
2. Add the onions and sauté until translucent, about 2-3 minutes.
3. Add the red and green bell peppers, and cook for another 3-4 minutes until slightly softened.
4. Stir in the crumbled tofu and spinach. Cook for 5 minutes, stirring occasionally.

5. Sprinkle in the turmeric, black pepper, salt (if using), and garlic powder. Mix well to combine all the ingredients evenly.

6. Continue to cook for another 5-7 minutes, until everything is heated through and the spinach is wilted.

7. Remove from heat and stir in the nutritional yeast. Adjust seasoning to taste.

Nutritional Information (per serving):

- Calories: 150
- Protein: 12 g
- Fat: 10 g
- Carbohydrates: 8 g
- Fiber: 3 g
- Sodium: 120 mg (varies if salt is added)

Serving Size: Serves 2

Cooking Time: Approximately 20 minutes

Quinoa Porridge with Almonds

Ingredients:
- 1 cup quinoa, rinsed
- 2 cups water
- 1/2 cup unsweetened almond milk
- 1/4 teaspoon cinnamon
- 1/2 teaspoon vanilla extract
- 1 tablespoon almond butter
- 1/4 cup slivered almonds
- 1 tablespoon chia seeds
- Optional: sweetener of choice (stevia or a sugar substitute suitable for diabetes)

Instructions:
1. Combine quinoa and water in a medium saucepan. Bring to a boil over high heat.
2. Reduce heat to low, cover, and simmer until the quinoa is tender and most of the water has been absorbed, about 15 minutes.
3. Stir in almond milk, cinnamon, and vanilla extract. Cook for another 5 minutes, stirring occasionally, until the mixture is creamy.

4. Remove from heat and stir in almond butter until well combined.

5. Serve the porridge topped with slivered almonds and chia seeds. Add a sweetener if desired.

Nutritional Information (per serving):

- Calories: 280
- Protein: 9g
- Carbohydrates: 38g
- Fiber: 6g
- Sugar: 1g (natural sugars from ingredients)
- Fat: 10g
- Sodium: 30mg

Serving Size: 1 cup

Cooking Time: 20 minutes

Apple Cinnamon Overnight Oats

Ingredients:

- 1/2 cup rolled oats
- 1 small apple, peeled and diced
- 1 tablespoon chia seeds
- 1/2 teaspoon ground cinnamon
- 1 tablespoon sugar-free maple syrup or sweetener of choice
- 3/4 cup unsweetened almond milk
- Optional toppings: chopped nuts, a sprinkle of ground flaxseed

Instructions:

1. In a mason jar or airtight container, combine the rolled oats, chia seeds, and ground cinnamon.
2. Add the diced apple and drizzle the sugar-free maple syrup over the top.
3. Pour the unsweetened almond milk into the jar, ensuring that all the ingredients are fully immersed.
4. Stir the mixture well, then seal the container and refrigerate overnight, or for at least 6 hours.
5. In the morning, give the oats a good stir. If the consistency is too thick, add a little more almond milk to achieve your desired thickness.

6. Serve cold, topped with optional nuts or a sprinkle of ground flaxseed for added texture and nutritional benefits.

Nutritional Information (per serving):
- Calories: 235
- Protein: 6 grams
- Fat: 7 grams
- Carbohydrates: 38 grams
- Fiber: 8 grams
- Sugar: 10 grams

Serving Size: 1 serving

Cooking Time: No cooking required; prepare in 5 minutes, ready to eat after refrigeration overnight.

Chapter 2: Lunch Recipes

Grilled Chicken Salad

Ingredients:

- 2 boneless, skinless chicken breasts
- 1 tbsp olive oil
- 1 tsp garlic powder
- 1/2 tsp ground black pepper
- 4 cups mixed greens (lettuce, spinach, arugula)
- 1/2 cup cherry tomatoes, halved
- 1/4 cup sliced cucumber
- 1/4 cup shredded carrots
- 2 tbsp red onion, thinly sliced
- 1/4 cup reduced-fat feta cheese, crumbled
- 2 tbsp balsamic vinegar
- 1 tbsp extra virgin olive oil
- 1/4 tsp dried oregano

Instructions:

1. Preheat grill to medium-high heat.

2. Rub the chicken breasts with olive oil, garlic powder, and black pepper.
3. Grill the chicken for 5-7 minutes on each side, or until fully cooked and internal temperature reaches 165°F.
4. Remove from grill and let rest for a few minutes. Slice thinly.
5. In a large bowl, combine mixed greens, cherry tomatoes, cucumber, carrots, and red onion.
6. Top the salad with sliced grilled chicken and crumbled feta cheese.
7. In a small bowl, whisk together balsachemical vinegar, extra virgin olive oil, and dried oregano. Drizzle over the salad.
8. Toss gently to combine and serve immediately.

Nutritional Information (per serving):
- Calories: 290
- Protein: 28 g
- Carbohydrates: 8 g
- Fat: 16 g
- Sodium: 320 mg
- Fiber: 2 g

Serving Size: 2 servings

Cooking Time: 15 minutes prep time + 14 minutes cooking time

Quinoa and Black Bean Bowl

Ingredients:

- 1 cup quinoa, rinsed
- 2 cups water
- 1 can (15 oz) low-sodium black beans, drained and rinsed
- 1 medium red bell pepper, diced
- 1/4 cup fresh cilantro, finely chopped
- 1/4 cup lime juice
- 1 tablespoon olive oil
- 1/2 teaspoon ground cumin
- Salt and pepper to taste (use sparingly if needed)
- 1 avocado, peeled, pitted, and diced
- 1/2 cup cherry tomatoes, halved

Instructions:

1. In a medium saucepan, combine the quinoa and water. Bring to a boil over high heat. Once boiling, reduce the heat to low, cover, and simmer until the quinoa is tender and the water is absorbed, about 15 to 20 minutes.
2. While the quinoa cooks, prepare the black beans, red bell pepper, cilantro, lime juice, olive oil, and cumin in a large bowl. Mix well to combine.

3. Once the quinoa is cooked, fluff it with a fork and let it cool slightly. Add the quinoa to the bowl with the bean mixture. Toss well to combine all the ingredients.

4. Gently fold in the avocado and cherry tomatoes. Adjust seasoning with salt and pepper, if needed.

5. Serve immediately or chill in the refrigerator before serving to enhance the flavors.

Nutritional Information (per serving):

- Calories: 320
- Protein: 12 g
- Fat: 10 g
- Carbohydrates: 46 g
- Fiber: 9 g
- Sodium: 30 mg
- Sugar: 3 g

Serving Size: 1 cup
Cooking Time: 20 minutes

Lentil Soup with Vegetables

Ingredients:

- 1 cup dried lentils, rinsed
- 1 large carrot, diced
- 1 stalk celery, diced
- 1 small onion, finely chopped
- 2 cloves garlic, minced
- 1 teaspoon olive oil
- 4 cups low-sodium vegetable broth
- 1 teaspoon ground cumin
- 1/2 teaspoon ground coriander
- 1/2 teaspoon dried thyme
- Salt and black pepper, to taste
- 2 cups spinach leaves, roughly chopped
- 1 tablespoon lemon juice

Instructions:

1. Heat the olive oil in a large pot over medium heat. Add the onions, carrots, and celery. Cook, stirring occasionally, until the vegetables are softened, about 5 minutes.
2. Add the garlic, cumin, coriander, and thyme. Cook for an additional minute until fragrant.

3. Stir in the rinsed lentils and vegetable broth. Bring to a boil, then reduce heat to low and simmer uncovered for about 25 minutes, or until the lentils are tender.
4. Add the chopped spinach and continue to simmer for 5 minutes.
5. Remove from heat and stir in lemon juice. Season with salt and pepper to taste.
6. Serve hot.

Nutritional Information (per serving):
- Calories: 210
- Protein: 14 g
- Carbohydrates: 35 g
- Fiber: 15 g
- Sodium: 120 mg
- Fat: 3 g

Serving Size: 1 bowl (approximately 1.5 cups)

Cooking Time: 35 minutes

Turkey and Avocado Wrap

Ingredients:
- 1 whole wheat tortilla (8-inch)
- 2 oz low-sodium turkey breast, thinly sliced
- 1/4 ripe avocado, thinly sliced
- 1/2 cup fresh spinach leaves
- 1 tablespoon hummus
- 1 small tomato, sliced
- 1/4 cucumber, sliced
- 1/4 teaspoon black pepper

Instructions:
1. Lay the tortilla flat on a clean surface. Spread the hummus evenly over the tortilla.
2. Arrange the turkey slices across the center of the tortilla.
3. Place the spinach leaves on top of the turkey.
4. Add the avocado, tomato, and cucumber slices over the spinach.
5. Sprinkle black pepper over the fillings.
6. Carefully fold the tortilla over the fillings, tucking in the edges as you roll to secure the wrap.
7. Cut the wrap in half diagonally.

Nutritional Information:

- Calories: 320
- Protein: 18 g
- Fat: 15 g
- Carbohydrates: 27 g
- Fiber: 6 g
- Sodium: 200 mg

Serving Size: 1 wrap

Cooking Time: 10 minutes (preparation time, no cooking required)

Chickpea Salad with Cucumber

Ingredients:

- 1 can (15 ounces) chickpeas, rinsed and drained
- 1 large cucumber, diced
- 1 red bell pepper, diced
- 1/4 cup red onion, finely chopped
- 2 tablespoons fresh parsley, chopped
- 1 tablespoon olive oil
- 2 tablespoons lemon juice
- 1/4 teaspoon garlic powder
- Salt (optional) and pepper to taste

Instructions:

1. In a large bowl, combine the chickpeas, cucumber, red bell pepper, red onion, and parsley.
2. In a small bowl, whisk together olive oil, lemon Joe, garlic powder, and a pinch of pepper. If your diet permits, add a small pinch of salt.
3. Pour the dressing over the salad and toss to coat evenly.
4. Refrigerate the salad for at least 30 minutes to allow flavors to blend. Serve chilled.

Nutritional Information (per serving):
- Calories: 180
- Protein: 6 g
- Carbohydrates: 24 g
- Fat: 7 g
- Sodium: 200 mg (varies if salt is added)
- Fiber: 6 g

Serving Size: 1 cup

Cooking Time: 10 minutes preparation, 30 minutes chilling

Spinach and Feta Stuffed Peppers

Ingredients:
- 4 large bell peppers, tops cut away and seeds removed
- 2 cups fresh spinach, chopped
- 1 cup crumbled feta cheese
- 1/2 cup cooked quinoa
- 1/4 cup onions, finely chopped
- 2 cloves garlic, minced
- 1 teaspoon olive oil
- 1/2 teaspoon dried oregano
- Salt and pepper to taste

Instructions:
1. Preheat your oven to 350°F (175°C).
2. In a skillet over medium heat, heat the olive use to sauté onions and garlic until translucent, about 3-4 minutes.
3. Add the spinach to the skillet and cook until it wilts, about 2 minutes. Remove from heat.
4. In a large bowl, combine the sautéed spinach and onions, cooked quinoa, feta cheese, oregano, salt, and pepper. Mix well.
5. Stuff each bell pepper with the spinach and feta mixture, packing it tightly.
6. Place the stuffed peppers upright in a baking dish and cover loosely with aluminum foil.

7. Bake in the preheated oven for about 30 minutes. Remove the foil and bake for an additional 10 minutes, or until the peppers are tender and the tops are slightly golden.

8. Serve warm.

Nutritional Information (per serving):

- Calories: 200
- Protein: 9 g
- Carbohydrates: 22 g
- Fat: 9 g
- Sodium: 320 mg
- Potassium: 349 mg
- Phosphorus: 120 mg
- Fiber: 4 g
- Sugar: 6 g

Serving Size: 1 stuffed pepper

Cooking Time: 40 minutes

Broccoli and Cheese Quiche (Low-Sodium)

Ingredients:

- 1 pre-made pie crust (low-sodium)
- 1 cup fresh broccoli florets, chopped
- 1 cup shredded cheddar cheese (low-fat)
- 4 large eggs
- 1 cup low-fat milk
- 1/2 teaspoon black pepper
- 1/4 teaspoon garlic powder

Instructions:

1. Preheat your oven to 350°F (175°C).
2. Arrange the pie crust in a 9-inch pie pan and set aside.
3. Blanch the broccoli florets in boiling water for 2 minutes, then drain and scatter evenly over the pie crust.
4. Sprinkle the shredded cheese over the broccoli.
5. In a mixing bowl, whisk together the eggs, milk, black an garlic powder until well combined.
6. Pour the egg mixture over the broccoli and cheese in the pie crust.
7. Bake in the preheated oven for 35 to 40 minutes, or until the center is set and the top is lightly golden.

8. Let the quiche rest for 10 minutes before slicing.

Nutritional Information (per serving):

- Calories: 220
- Total Fat: 12g (Saturated Fat: 5g)
- Cholesterol: 125mg
- Sodium: 180mg
- Total Carbohydrates: 16g (Dietary Fiber: 2g, Total Sugars: 3g)
- Protein: 12g

Serving Size: 1 slice

Cooking Time: 40 minutes

Total Time: 50 minutes (includes preparation and cooling)

Tuna Salad with Olive Oil Dressing

Ingredients:

- 1 can (5 ounces) of tuna, packed in water, drained
- 1/4 cup red onion, finely chopped
- 1/4 cup celery, finely chopped
- 2 tablespoons fresh parsley, chopped
- 1/4 cup cucumber, chopped
- 2 tablespoons extra virgin olive oil
- 1 tablespoon lemon juice
- Salt and pepper to taste (use minimal salt if advised for CKD and diabetes management)
- Lettuce leaves or mixed greens for serving

Instructions:

1. In a mixing bowl, combine the drained tuna, red onion, celery, parsley, and cucumber.
2. In a small separate bowl, whisk together the olive oil and lemon juice. Add a pinch of salt and pepper to taste. Remember to keep salt minimal due to dietary restrictions.
3. Pour the dressing over the tuna mixture and toss gently until well combined.
4. Chill the salad in the refrigerator for at least 30 minutes to allow the flavors to meld.
5. Serve on a bed of lettuce leaves or mixed greens.

Nutritional Information:
- Calories: 220 per serving
- Protein: 25 g
- Carbohydrates: 4 g
- Dietary Fiber: 1 g
- Sugars: 2 g
- Fat: 12 g
- Sodium: 190 mg (check with a dietitian for modifications if sodium intake is a concern)

Serving Size:
- Makes 2 servings.

Cooking Time:
- Preparation time: 10 minutes
- Chill time: 30 minutes

Baked Salmon with Asparagus

Ingredients:

- 4 salmon fillets (6 ounces each)
- 1 bunch of asparagus, trimmed
- 2 tablespoons olive oil
- 1 teaspoon garlic powder
- Salt (optional) and pepper to taste
- 1 lemon, sliced
- Fresh dill for garnish

Instructions:

1. Preheat the oven to 400°F (200°C).
2. Arrange the salmon fillets and asparagus on a baking sheet lined with parchment paper for easy cleanup.
3. Brush the salmon and asparagus with olive oil. Sprinkle garlic powder, and pepper over both. If using salt, do so sparingly as both CKD and diabetes require low sodium intake.
4. Top each salmon fillet with a couple of lemon slices.
5. Bake in the preheated oven for 15-20 minutes, or until the salmon is opaque and flakes easily with a fork and the asparagus is tender.
6. Remove from oven and garnish with fresh dill before serving.

Nutritional Information per serving:

- Calories: 295
- Protein: 34 g
- Fat: 16 g (Saturated Fat: 3 g)
- Carbohydrates: 5 g
- Fiber: 2 g
- Sodium: 50 mg (note this may vary if salt is added)

Serving Size: 1 salmon fillet with a portion of asparagus

Cooking Time: 20 minutes

Veggie Stir-Fry with Tofu

Ingredients:

- 1 block firm tofu (14 ounces), pressed and cut into cubes
- 2 tablespoons olive oil
- 1 cup broccoli florets
- 1 cup sliced bell peppers (mix of red, yellow, and green)
- 1/2 cup sliced carrots
- 1/2 cup snow peas
- 2 cloves garlic, minced
- 1 tablespoon ginger, freshly grated
- 2 tablespoons low-sodium soy sauce
- 1 tablespoon sesame oil
- 1 teaspoon cornstarch (optional, for thickening)
- Fresh cilantro, chopped (for garnish)
- Sesame seeds (for garnish)

Instructions:

1. In a non-stick skillet, heat 1 tablespoon olive oil over medium-high heat. Add tofu cubes and sauté until golden brown on all sides, about 7-10 minutes. Remove from skillet and set aside.
2. In the same skillet, add the remaining olive oil. Sauté garlic and ginger for 1 minute until fragrant. Add broccoli, bell peppers,

carrots, and snow peas. Stir-fry for about 5 minutes or until vegetables are just tender.

3. Return the tofu to the skillet with the vegetables. Drizzle with soy sauce and sesame oil, stirring gently to combine.

4. If a thicker sauce is desired, mix cornstarch with 2 tablespoons of water and stir into the skillet. Cook for another 2 minutes until the sauce is slightly thickened.

5. Remove from heat. Sprinkle with chopped cilantro and sesame seeds before serving.

Nutritional Information (per serving):

- Calories: 280
- Protein: 18 g
- Carbohydrates: 20 g
- Fat: 15 g
- Sodium: 350 mg
- Fiber: 4 g

Serving Size: 1 bowl (approximately 1.5 cups)

Cooking Time: 20 minutes

Chapter 3: Dinner Recipes

Baked Chicken with Rosemary

Ingredients:

- 4 boneless, skinless chicken breasts
- 2 tablespoons olive oil
- 2 cloves garlic, minced
- 1 tablespoon fresh rosemary, finely chopped
- 1 teaspoon lemon zest
- 1/2 teaspoon black pepper
- 1/4 teaspoon salt (optional, based on dietary needs)
- 1 lemon, sliced into rounds for garnish

Instructions:

1. Preheat the oven to 375°F (190°C).
2. In a small bowl, mix together the olive oil, garlic, rosemary, lemon zest, black pepper, and salt if using.
3. Place the chicken breasts in a baking dish. Rub the olive oil and herb mixture over both sides of the chicken.
4. Arrange lemon slices on and around the chicken in the dish.

5. Bake in the preheated oven for 25 to 30 minutes, or until the chicken is thoroughly cooked and reaches an internal temperature of 165°F (74°C).

6. Remove from the oven and let rest for 5 minutes before serving to allow the juices to redistribute.

Nutritional Information (per serving):

- Calories: 230
- Protein: 26 g
- Total Fat: 13 g (Saturated Fat: 2 g)
- Carbohydrates: 2 g
- Fiber: 0.5 g
- Sodium: 150 mg (varies if salt is omitted)

Serving Size: 1 chicken breast

Cooking Time: 30 minutes

Beef and Vegetable Stew

Ingredients:

- 1 pound beef chuck, cut into 1-inch cubes
- 2 tablespoons olive oil
- 2 medium carrots, peeled and diced
- 2 celery stalks, diced
- 1 small onion, diced
- 2 cloves garlic, minced
- 1 medium zucchini, diced
- 1 cup green beans, trimmed and cut into 1-inch pieces
- 1 teaspoon dried thyme
- 1 bay leaf
- 4 cups low-sodium beef broth
- Salt (optional) and pepper to taste
- 2 tablespoons chopped fresh parsley

Instructions:

1. Heat the olive oil in a large pot over medium heat. Add the beef cubes and brown on all sides, about 5-7 minutes. Remove the beef and set aside.
2. In the same pot, add onions, carrots, and celery. Cook until vegetables are softened, about 5 minutes. Add garlic and cook for an additional minute.

3. Return the beef to the pot along with zucchini, green beans, thyme, and bay leaf. Pour in the beef broth and bring to a boil.
4. Reduce heat to a simmer and cover. Cook for about 1-1.5 hours or until the beef is tender.
5. Adjust seasoning with salt (if using) and pepper. Remove the bay leaf and discard.
6. Garnish with fresh parsley before serving.

Nutritional Information per serving:
- Calories: 250
- Protein: 26g
- Carbohydrates: 15g
- Fiber: 4g
- Sugar: 5g
- Fat: 10g
- Sodium: 150mg (varies if salt is added)

Serving Size: 1 cup

Cooking Time: Approximately 1 hour 45 minutes

Grilled Shrimp with Zucchini Noodles

Ingredients:

- 1 lb large shrimp, peeled and deveined
- 2 large zucchinis
- 1 tablespoon olive oil
- 1 teaspoon garlic powder
- 1/2 teaspoon smoked paprika
- Salt and pepper to taste
- 1 lemon, for garnish
- Fresh parsley, chopped (for garnish)

Instructions:

1. Preheat the grill to medium-high heat.
2. Using a spiralizer, turn the zucchinis into noodles. Set aside.
3. In a large bowl, mix the olive oil, garlic powder, smoked paprika, salt, and pepper. Add the shrimp and toss to coat evenly.
4. Thread the shrimp onto skewers. If using wooden skewers, soak them in water for 30 minutes beforehand to prevent burning.
5. Grill the shrimp for 2-3 minutes on each side, or until they are pink and opaque.
6. While the shrimp cooks, heat a non-stick skillet over medium heat. Add the zucchini noodles and sauté for 2-3 minutes until tender but still firm.

7. Serve the grilled shrimp over the bed of zucchini noodles. Garnish with fresh parsley and a squeeze of lemon juice.

Nutritional Information (per serving):
- Calories: 200
- Protein: 24 g
- Carbohydrates: 6 g
- Fiber: 2 g
- Fat: 10 g
- Sodium: 320 mg
- Cholesterol: 180 mg

Serving Size: 4 servings

Cooking Time: 10 minutes preparation, 6 minutes cooking

Stuffed Bell Peppers with Quinoa

Ingredients:
- 4 large bell peppers, tops cut, seeded
- 1 cup quinoa, cooked
- 1 tablespoon olive oil
- 1/2 cup onion, finely chopped
- 2 cloves garlic, minced
- 1/2 cup tomatoes, diced
- 1/4 cup carrots, finely diced
- 1/4 cup celery, finely diced
- 1/2 teaspoon cumin
- 1 teaspoon dried oregano
- 1/4 cup fresh parsley, chopped
- Salt and pepper to taste (use minimal salt for CKD and diabetes management)
- 1/4 cup low-sodium cheese (optional), shredded

Instructions:
1. Preheat the oven to 375°F (190°C).
2. In a skillet, heat the olive oil over medium heat. Add onions and garlic, sauté until onions are translucent.
3. Stir in tomatoes, carrots, and celery; cook for about 5 minutes until vegetables are softened.

4. Mix in the cooked quinoa, cumin, oregano, parsley, salt, and pepper. Cook together for another 2-3 minutes.
5. Fill each bell pepper with the quinoa mixture and place them in a baking dish.
6. If using cheese, sprinkle the tops of the stuffed peppers with shredded cheese.
7. Bake in the preheated oven for 25-30 minutes, until peppers are tender and the filling is heated through.

Nutritional Information (per serving):

- Calories: 200
- Total Fat: 5g
- Saturated Fat: 1g
- Cholesterol: 0mg
- Sodium: 50mg
- Total Carbohydrates: 35g
- Dietary Fiber: 6g
- Sugars: 8g
- Protein: 8g

Serving Size: 1 stuffed pepper

Cooking Time: 30 minutes

Eggplant Parmesan (Low-Sodium)

Ingredients:

- 1 large eggplant, sliced into 1/2-inch thick rounds
- 2 eggs, beaten
- 1 cup almond flour
- 1/2 cup grated Parmesan cheese (low-sodium)
- 1 tsp garlic powder
- 1 tsp dried basil
- 2 cups low-sodium marinara sauce
- 1 cup shredded mozzarella cheese (low-moisture, part-skim)
- Fresh basil leaves, for garnish
- Olive oil spray

Instructions:

1. Preheat your oven to 375°F (190°C). Line a baking sheet with parchment paper and lightly spray with olive oil.
2. In a shallow dish, mix almond flour, grated Parmesan, garlic powder, and dried basil.
3. Dip each eggplant slice in the beaten eggs, then dredge in the almond flour mixture, coating evenly.
4. Place coated eggplant slices on the prepared baking sheet and spray the tops lightly with olive oil.
5. Bake in the preheated oven for 20-25 minutes, flipping halfway through, until golden and crispy.

6. In a baking dish, spread a thin layer of marinara sauce. Layer half of the baked eggplant slices over the sauce. Spoon more marinara over the eggplant and sprinkle with half of the mozzarella cheese.

7. Repeat layers with remaining eggplant, marinara, and mozzarella.

8. Bake in the oven for 20-25 minutes, or until the cheese is bubbly and golden.

9. Garnish with fresh basil leaves before serving.

Nutritional Information (per serving):

- Calories: 320
- Total Fat: 18g
- Saturated Fat: 6g
- Cholesterol: 90mg
- Sodium: 340mg
- Total Carbohydrates: 24g
- Dietary Fiber: 8g
- Sugars: 8g
- Protein: 18g

Serving Size: 1 slice

Cooking Time: 45-50 minutes

Roasted Turkey Breast with Brussels Sprouts

Ingredients:

- 1 lb turkey breast, boneless and skinless
- 1 lb Brussels sprouts, trimmed and halved
- 2 tbsp olive oil
- 1 tsp dried thyme
- 1 tsp garlic powder
- Salt and pepper, to taste

Instructions:

1. Preheat your oven to 375°F (190°C).
2. In a large mixing bowl, toss the Brussels sprouts with 1 tablespoon of olive oil, salt, and pepper.
3. Spread the Brussels sprouts on one half of a baking sheet.
4. In the same bowl, add the remaining olive oil, thyme, garlic powder, salt, and pepper. Add the turkey breast and coat evenly with the seasoning.
5. Place the seasoned turkey breast on the other half of the baking sheet.
6. Roast in the preheated oven for 25-30 minutes, or until the turkey is thoroughly cooked (internal temperature should reach 165°F) and the Brussels sprouts are tender and caramelized.

7. Remove from oven and let the turkey rest for a few minutes before slicing.

Nutritional Information (per serving):
- Calories: 295
- Protein: 38g
- Carbohydrates: 11g
- Fat: 12g
- Fiber: 4g
- Sodium: 220mg

Serving Size: 4 servings

Cooking Time: 30 minutes

Pork Tenderloin with Apples

Ingredients:
- 1 lb pork tenderloin
- 2 apples, peeled, cored, and sliced
- 1 small onion, thinly sliced
- 2 cloves garlic, minced
- 1/4 cup apple cider vinegar
- 1 tablespoon olive oil
- 1 teaspoon dried thyme
- 1/2 teaspoon ground cinnamon
- Salt and pepper to taste
- Fresh parsley, chopped (for garnish)

Instructions:
1. Preheat the oven to 375°F (190°C).
2. Heat olive oil in a large ovenproof skillet over medium heat. Season the pork tenderloin with salt, pepper, thyme, and cinnamon.
3. Sear the tenderloin until golden brown on all sides, about 2-3 minutes per side.
4. Remove the tenderloin from the skillet and set aside. In the same skillet, add onion and garlic. Sauté until the onions are translucent.

5. Add the sliced apples to the skillet and cook for about 2 minutes until they start to soften.
6. Place the seared tenderloin back in the skillet with the apples and onions. Pour the apple cider vinegar over the pork.
7. Transfer the skillet to the oven and roast for 20-25 minutes, or until the pork reaches an internal temperature of 145°F (63°C).
8. Let the pork rest for a few minutes before slicing. Serve garnished with fresh parsley.

Nutritional Information (per serving):

- Calories: 220
- Protein: 24 g
- Fat: 7 g
- Carbohydrates: 15 g
- Fiber: 3 g
- Sodium: 65 mg

Serving Size: 4 oz pork with a quarter of the apple and onion mixture

Cooking Time: 30-35 minutes (Preparation: 10 minutes, Cooking: 20-25 minutes)

Spaghetti Squash with Tomato Sauce

Ingredients:

- 1 medium spaghetti squash
- 2 tablespoons olive oil
- 1/2 teaspoon salt (optional, to taste)
- 1/4 teaspoon black pepper
- 1 clove garlic, minced
- 1 small onion, finely chopped
- 1 can (14 ounces) no-salt-added diced tomatoes
- 1 teaspoon dried basil
- 1 teaspoon dried oregano
- 1/4 cup fresh basil, chopped (for garnish)

Instructions:

1. Preheat the oven to 400°F (204°C). Halve the spaghetti squash lengthwise and scoop out the seeds.
2. Drizzle the inside of each half with 1 tablespoon of olive oil and season with pepper, and salt if using. Place the squash halves cut-side down on a baking sheet and roast in the oven for 40 minutes, or until the flesh is tender and easily shreds with a fork.
3. While the squash is roasting, heat the remaining tablespoon of olive oil in a saucepan over medium heat. Add the garlic and onion, sautéing until the onion becomes translucent, about 5 minutes.

4. Stir in the diced tomatoes, dried basil, and oregano. Bring the mixture to a simmer and cook for 10 minutes, allowing the flavors to meld.
5. Once the squash is done, use a fork to shred the inside flesh into spaghetti-like strands, leaving the shell intact.
6. Spoon the tomato sauce over the spaghetti squash strands and garnish with fresh basil.

Nutritional Information (per serving):

- Calories: 150
- Total Fat: 7g
- Saturated Fat: 1g
- Cholesterol: 0mg
- Sodium: 50mg (without added salt)
- Total Carbohydrates: 22g
- Dietary Fiber: 5g
- Sugars: 8g
- Protein: 3g

Serving Size: 1/2 of a medium squash filled with sauce

Cooking Time: Approximately 55 minutes (15 minutes preparation time + 40 minutes cooking time)

Cod Fillet with Green Beans

Ingredients:

- 4 cod fillets (6 ounces each)
- 2 tablespoons olive oil
- 1 teaspoon garlic powder
- Salt (to taste, optional)
- Black pepper (to taste)
- 1 pound green beans, trimmed
- 1 lemon, sliced into wedges
- 2 tablespoons fresh parsley, chopped (for garnish)

Instructions:

1. Preheat your oven to 400°F (200°C).
2. Arrange cod fillets on a greased baking sheet.
3. Brush each fillet with olive oil and sprinkle garlic powder, salt (if using), and black peeper evenly over the top.
4. Toss green beans in the remaining olive oil and season with a pinch of salt and pepper. Spread them around the cod on the baking sheet.
5. Bake in the preheated oven for 12-15 minutes, or until the cod flakes easily with a fork and green beans are tender-crisp.
6. Remove from oven and squeeze lemon wedges over the cooked cod and green beans.
7. Garnish with fresh parsley before serving.

Nutritional Information:

- Calories: 220
- Total Fat: 10g
- Saturated Fat: 1.5g
- Cholesterol: 60mg
- Sodium: 70mg
- Total Carbohydrates: 9g (Dietary Fiber: 4g, Sugars: 3g)
- Protein: 27g

Serving Size: 1 fillet with a quarter of the green beans

Cooking Time: 12-15 minutes

Chickpea and Spinach Curry

Ingredients:

- 1 tablespoon olive oil
- 1 large onion, finely chopped
- 2 cloves garlic, minced
- 1 tablespoon ginger, freshly grated
- 1 tablespoon garam masala
- 1 teaspoon turmeric
- 1 teaspoon cumin
- 1/2 teaspoon coriander
- 1/4 teaspoon cayenne pepper (optional)
- 1 can (15 ounces) chickpeas, drained and rinsed
- 1 can (14 ounces) diced tomatoes, no salt added
- 4 cups fresh spinach leaves
- 1/2 cup light coconut milk
- Salt to taste (optional)

Instructions:

1. Heat olive oil in a large skillet over medium heat. Add onion, garlic, and ginger, cooking until the onion is translucent, about 5 minutes.
2. Stir in garam masala, turmeric, cumin, coriander, and cayenne pepper. Cook for 1 minute until fragrant.

3. Add chickpeas and diced tomatoes with their juice. Bring to a simmer, then reduce heat and cook for 10 minutes, allowing the flavors to meld.
4. Add spinach and cover the skillet. Let it sit for 2-3 minutes or until the spinach is wilted.
5. Stir in the coconut milk and continue to cook for another 5 minutes, until the curry is heated through and slightly thickened. Adjust seasoning with salt if needed.
6. Remove from heat and serve warm.

Nutritional Information:

- Calories: 250 per serving
- Total Fat: 8g
- Saturated Fat: 3g
- Cholesterol: 0mg
- Sodium: 300mg (varies with added salt)
- Total Carbohydrates: 35g
- Dietary Fiber: 9g
- Sugars: 7g
- Protein: 9g

Serving Size: 1 cup

Cooking Time: 25 minutes

Chapter 4: Snacks and Desserts

Healthy Snack Options

Apple Cinnamon Yogurt Bowl

Ingredients:
- 1 small apple, peeled and chopped
- 1 cup low-fat Greek yogurt
- 1/4 teaspoon ground cinnamon
- 1 tablespoon chopped walnuts (optional)

Instructions:
1. Mix the Greek yogurt with ground cinnamon in a bowl.
2. Top with chopped apple and walnuts if using.
3. Serve immediately or chill for 30 minutes for enhanced flavors.

Nutritional Information:
- Calories: 150
- Carbohydrates: 18g
- Protein: 12g
- Fat: 2g
- Sodium: 55mg
- Potassium: 210mg

Serving Size: 1 bowl

Cooking Time: 5 minutes

Carrot and Hummus Dip

Ingredients:
- 2 medium carrots, peeled and cut into sticks
1/3 cup low-sodium hummus

Instructions:
1. Peel and cut carrots into stick-sized pieces.
2. Serve with a side of low-sodium hummus for dipping.

Nutritional Information:
- Calories: 135
- Carbohydrates: 20g
- Protein: 6g
- Fat: 4.5g
- Sodium: 210mg
- Potassium: 320mg

Serving Size: 1 serving
Cooking Time: 10 minutes

Healthy Dessert Options

Berry Almond Crisp

Ingredients:
- 1 cup fresh mixed berries (blueberries, raspberries)
- 2 tablespoons sliced almonds
- 1 tablespoon almond flour
- 1 tablespoon unsalted butter, melted
- 1/4 teaspoon vanilla extract

Instructions:
1. Preheat oven to 350°F.
2. In a baking dish, layer the berries and sprinkle with almond flour and almonds.
3. Drizzle melted butter and vanilla extract over the top.
4. Bake for 15-20 minutes until the topping is golden and berries are bubbly.

Nutritional Information:
- Calories: 185
- Carbohydrates: 15g
- Protein: 4g
- Fat: 12g
- Sodium: 5mg
- Potassium: 105mg

Serving Size: 1/2 cup
Cooking Time: 20 minutes

Chia Pudding with Kiwi

Ingredients:
- 2 tablespoons chia seeds
- 1/2 cup unsweetened almond milk
- 1 kiwi, peeled and sliced
- 1 teaspoon honey (optional)

Instructions:
1. In a bowl, combine chia seeds with almond milk and honey if using. Stir well.
2. Refrigerate for at least 4 hours or overnight until the mixture achieves a pudding-like consistency.
3. Top with fresh kiwi slices before serving.

Nutritional Information:
- Calories: 150
- Carbohydrates: 21g
- Protein: 5g
- Fat: 7g
- Sodium: 30mg
- Potassium: 285mg

Serving Size: 1 bowl
Cooking Time: 4 hours (mostly refrigeration time)

These snack and dessert options are specifically designed to be kidney and blood sugar-friendly, catering to the dietary needs of individuals with CKD Stage 3 and Diabetes Type 2.

Diabetes-Friendly Desserts

Apple Cinnamon Greek Yogurt Parfait

Ingredients:
- 1 cup plain Greek yogurt
- 1 medium apple, diced
- 1/2 teaspoon ground cinnamon
- 1 tablespoon honey (optional)
- 1/4 cup walnuts, chopped

Instructions:
1. In a bowl, mix the diced apple with cinnamon.
2. Layer half the Greek yogurt in a serving glass.
3. Add half of the apple-cinnamon mixture.
4. Repeat the layers with the remaining yogurt and apples.
5. Top with chopped walnuts and a drizzle of honey if desired.

Nutritional Information (per serving):
- Calories: 200
- Carbohydrates: 25g
- Protein: 15g
- Fat: 7g
- Sodium: 60mg

- Potassium: 300mg
- Phosphorus: 200mg

Serving Size: 1 parfait
Cooking Time: 10 minutes

Berry Chia Seed Pudding

Ingredients:
- 1/4 cup chia seeds
- 1 cup unsweetened almond milk
- 1 teaspoon vanilla extract
- 1 cup mixed berries (strawberries, blueberries, raspberries)
- 1 tablespoon stevia or monk fruit sweetener (optional)

Instructions:
1. In a bowl, whisk together chia seeds, almond milk, and vanilla extract.
2. Cover and refrigerate for at least 4 hours or overnight until thickened.
3. Stir the pudding to break up any clumps.
4. Divide the pudding into serving bowls and top with mixed berries.
5. Add sweetener if desired.

Nutritional Information (per serving):

- Calories: 150
- Carbohydrates: 20g
- Protein: 5g
- Fat: 8g
- Sodium: 50mg
- Potassium: 180mg
- Phosphorus: 100mg

Serving Size: 2 servings
Cooking Time: 4 hours (chilling time)

Peanut Butter Banana Bites

Ingredients:
- 2 bananas, sliced into rounds
- 1/4 cup natural peanut butter
- 2 tablespoons unsweetened cocoa powder
- 1 tablespoon coconut oil, melted

Instructions:
1. Spread a small amount of peanut butter on each banana slice.
2. Sandwich another banana slice on top to create a mini sandwich.
3. In a small bowl, mix cocoa powder and melted coconut oil until smooth.
4. Dip each banana sandwich halfway into the chocolate mixture.

5. Place the bites on a parchment-lined tray and refrigerate until the chocolate sets.

Nutritional Information (per serving):
- Calories: 180
- Carbohydrates: 25g
- Protein: 4g
- Fat: 9g
- Sodium: 40mg
- Potassium: 350mg
- Phosphorus: 70mg

Serving Size: 4 bites
Cooking Time: 20 minutes

Almond Flour Chocolate Chip Cookies

Ingredients:
- 2 cups almond flour
- 1/4 cup coconut oil, melted
- 1/4 cup stevia or monk fruit sweetener
- 1 teaspoon vanilla extract
- 1/2 teaspoon baking soda
- 1/2 cup sugar-free chocolate chips

Instructions:

1. Preheat oven to 350°F (175°C).
2. In a large bowl, mix almond flour, coconut oil, sweetener, vanilla extract, and baking soda until well combined.
3. Fold in chocolate chips.
4. Drop spoonfuls of dough onto a parchment-lined baking sheet.
5. Flatten each cookie slightly with a fork.
6. Bake for 10-12 minutes or until edges are golden brown.

Nutritional Information (per cookie):

- Calories: 150
- Carbohydrates: 8g
- Protein: 4g
- Fat: 12g
- Sodium: 70mg
- Potassium: 40mg
- Phosphorus: 60mg

Serving Size: 12 cookies
Cooking Time: 15 minutes

Conclusion

Managing CKD Stage 3 and Type 2 Diabetes can be challenging, but with the right dietary choices, it is possible to enjoy delicious, nutritious meals that support overall health and well-being. This cookbook has been designed to provide a variety of recipes tailored to meet the specific needs of individuals with these conditions. From hearty breakfasts to satisfying dinners, and from nutritious snacks to delectable desserts, each recipe focuses on balancing key nutrients while minimizing harmful components like excess sodium, potassium, and phosphorus.

By incorporating these recipes into your daily routine, you can enjoy flavorful meals that not only meet your dietary restrictions but also contribute to better blood sugar control and kidney function. The emphasis on whole foods, lean proteins, healthy fats, and low-glycemic carbohydrates ensures that each meal supports your body's needs without compromising on taste.

In addition to following these recipes, it's crucial to maintain regular communication with your healthcare provider and dietitian. They can provide personalized advice and adjustments based on your specific health status and needs. Remember, managing CKD and diabetes is a continuous process that involves careful monitoring, lifestyle adjustments, and a commitment to healthy eating.

This cookbook aims to empower you with practical and enjoyable meal options, helping you take control of your health journey. Whether you're new to cooking or an experienced home chef, these recipes are designed to be easy to follow, nutritious, and delicious. Embrace the variety and creativity in your kitchen, and discover how satisfying and healthful meals can enhance your quality of life.

Thank you for choosing this cookbook as a resource in your journey toward better health. May it serve as a helpful guide and inspiration for many enjoyable meals to come.

www.ingramcontent.com/pod-product-compliance
Lightning Source LLC
Chambersburg PA
CBHW050232230526
45470CB00005B/1913